~~WEIGHT~~ FAT LOSS

The Forbidden Secret to Weight Loss,
What No One Else Is Telling You

~~WEIGHT~~ FAT LOSS

Based on Weight Loss Research

DR. MARIA H.

Leany Bean Books

~~Weight~~ *Fat Loss* by Dr. Maria H. Published by Leany Bean Books

Leany Bean Books

www.leanybean.com

For permissions, contact:
info@leanybean.com

v1.4

DISCLAIMER

The material contained within this book is for informational purposes only. All efforts have been executed to present accurate, up-to-date, reliable, complete information. No warranties of any kind are declared or implied. Readers acknowledge that the author is not engaged in the rendering of legal, financial, medical, or professional advice. The content within this book has been derived from various sources. These opinions reflect the research and ideas of the author but are not intended to substitute for the services of a trained healthcare practitioner. As each individual's situation is unique, you should use proper discretion, in consultation with a health care practitioner, before undertaking the diet, exercises, and techniques described in this book. The testimonials and examples provided in this book show exceptional results, which may not apply to the average reader, and are not intended to represent or guarantee that you will achieve the same or similar results. The author and publisher expressly disclaim responsibility for any adverse effects resulting directly or indirectly from the use or application of the information contained in this book.

For my family, especially my husband

Without whose support this book wouldn't have been possible.

ABOUT THE AUTHOR

Fat loss expert Dr. Maria H. is a registered medical doctor and fitness enthusiast, currently in her post-graduate residency. She is happily married and lives with her husband in Lahore. Dr. Maria is also an avid reader, her hobbies include baking delicious cinnamon rolls and exploring new places. She also enjoys writing and the occasional shopping spree. In between juggling patients, hospital life, and home, Dr. Maria has managed to produce an amazing book that has changed the way people view health and fitness.

It was Dr. Maria's own passionate journey towards a sustainable healthier lifestyle that led her to research and test a fitness and health program that she developed for herself over the years. Starting out, she focused on her career and settled for quick fixes with regard to health, and as a result her health declined. Then, she relied on her knowledge, saw through the gimmicks, and created this program. The initiative gained popularity amongst her peers and soon extended to family and friends who were truly impressed with her phenomenal success. Dr. Maria went on to share her wisdom with more people.

With her medical background being the guiding light, Dr. Maria continued to fine-tune her incredible regime.

Her methods empower individuals to take ownership of their health and fitness, making wiser choices that will last a lifetime.

This book is a must-read for all health, fitness and weight loss seekers, wishing to make this their last fat loss journey.

Dr. Maria continues to dedicate her time and energy into researching and writing new ways to help health and fitness enthusiasts.

CONTENTS

~~WEIGHT~~ FAT LOSS

INTRODUCTION

We live in a world full of Instagram filters and Snapstreaks, where everything has a quick fix! It's increasingly difficult to tackle weight loss with the multitude of fad diets and tricks splattered over the Internet pulling and tugging at you from all directions.

"Why don't you join the gym!", one might say. But if you're reading this book right now, I'm quite sure you have tried some sort of exercise and activity to kickstart your dream 'weight loss' journey already. The real question is, did it lead you to the Kardashian cinched waist or a Mr. Dwayne Johnson inspired six pack yet? I'm guessing no.

Many of us have been through this frustration, where you give up and start to negotiate with yourself, rationalizing and saying, "well, this is just my bone weight," or, "I have just got a wider skeletal structure".

But to be honest, secretly you want to fit into your favorite dress or suit that you just put down after picking it up because you're thinking that your body will not look good in it. Hell, I'm guilty of it too! The wishing and sighing that comes with wanting to look good in whatever you want to wear! It is frustrating and taxing.

On the other hand, maybe it's not about the body image for you; maybe you're just looking to be healthy and stay fit.

Well, I'm here to tell you that if you're a fairly healthy and active individual, there is nothing stopping you from reaching your goal weight if you stick with me.

I know exactly what it is like. Personally, I have struggled through the tumultuous phase of yo-yo diets that bring you nothing but meme-ful disappointment! However, with my background knowledge as a doctor and the undying quest for fitness, together we will finally be able to crack the code on how to achieve sustainable weight loss minus the frustration!

Who knew being a compulsive note taker would come in handy someday? This book is basically the result of that researched-backed note taking that I developed for my own use. My initial intention was to keep these notes private and help our family, friends, colleagues, and clients. But one of my close friends convinced me to write it down in the form of a book so that it can reach and benefit people beyond the limited circle around me. That's how this book came into being.

WHY READ A BOOK ABOUT WEIGHT LOSS?

You might ask yourself, why read a book? How will that help me achieve my weight loss goals? This is exactly what came to my mind when I started to read about weight loss instead of those YouTube videos of Hollywood cardio training lined up on my watch list.

Basically, I was just tired of feeling helpless after gaining the pounds that I didn't even notice I was putting on. A snack here and there, fast food on the go, shakes or a Coke with every meal! And behold, slowly but surely the weight gain crept on me sneakily. Before I knew it, I wasn't fitting into my old jeans.

At first that doesn't seem like much, but over time you start to change your whole wardrobe, it starts to obstruct and alter your style. Eventually your whole personality is overshadowed by the few pounds that became many, and now you sit on your phone or laptop searching how to lose it overnight. Truth is, you didn't gain it overnight and you won't lose it overnight.

You try out those well schemed fad diets for a few days and give up, feeling frustrated and stuck while everyone else around you seems to know exactly how to shed their holiday weight. You're stuck thinking something might be wrong with you. The frustration leads to depression, and your hand reaches for another cookie for you to self soothe. But wait! Stop! We can change this!

I was there once too, but I broke that vicious cycle of self-harm and frustration. You'll be alright! I will help you discover the secret of how and what I found that helped me move smoothly on the journey. I learned why I wasn't achieving the same results as many other friends who seemed to know the secret.

Basically, weight loss is not a linear line as some of us tend to think. Losing inches on our waists or pounds on the scale is a process that has many variables. You won't achieve that model figure you dreamed of overnight. Without sound knowledge based on scientific principles, you will go in blind and set yourself up to not meet the expectations that you have.

With a doctorate degree under my belt and with a lot of professional and personal experience as a fitness enthusiast, I decided to jot down everything I discovered. That process led me to this book; to help people through what I was once stuck with! Even though there is no shortcut to weight loss, as Kylie's slim tea might suggest, there is definitely a well proven way that you can take to reach the finish line smoothly!

A good basic knowledge of what you are getting into will not only help you execute your plan better, but will also bring a great sense of achievement when you reach each of your smaller milestones.

Let's begin with the thought that weight loss is essentially a step into fitness and a healthier lifestyle rather than a plunge into unknown dark waters. Think of it as joining a fitness movement!

#TheLeanyBeanMovement

READ THIS FIRST – HOW TO USE THIS BOOK

When I started my own personal weight loss journey, as I have mentioned earlier, I was practically lost in a maze of information. I would go days without eating a full meal and then end up going on a binge that would take me back to where I began. Then, I moved on to joining the gym and putting all my money in a place hoping that it would somehow magically fix me. I would resort to buying from the most expensive lane in the super stores, from everything and anything that said low fat, low carb or diet! I would grab it and stockpile it in my kitchen. But all my effort would only get me a few pounds down at most, which would easily be gained back by a single weekend out. It is safe to say that my weight loss journey wasn't going smoothly because I failed to understand the basics of it.

The amount of information that bombarded me from this multi-billion-dollar weight loss industry was confusing and conflicting at best. I remember when I just wanted someone with a scientific background to sit me down and tell me exactly what is right or wrong. So I decided to be that person for myself. I gathered whatever knowledge came my way and made my own path. Even if I was lost for the most part in the beginning, I managed to pave a path, not just for myself, but for many others that I have led down this path of science-backed weight loss.

So, let me help you out of this maze by lending you a hand and lighting the way. My goal is to help you understand that diet management is essentially a process consisting of different stages and how you can go through them step-by-step.

For better understanding, I have divided this book in three sections that correspond to the phases one experiences on a weight loss journey. Each section focuses on a particular phase: *getting started, active weight loss,* and *stagnation* during your diet management program.

In the first part, 'The How,' we will go through the main mechanisms of fat loss and diet management and the basic nutritional make-up for your body.

The second part, 'The Help,' will shed some light on the role of exercise and activity on your weight loss journey.

The third part, 'The Halt,' we will be dealing with this necessary evil, *the plateau,* which I know is the biggest bummer in this whole process! But this miraculous section will tell what I learned the hard way, how to deal with this phase of your weight loss journey, and why it happens. So, let's get to it!

Disclaimer:

If you have a kidney, liver or any other serious disease consult with your doctor first before starting this regimen. Pregnant females are also not recommended to follow fat or weight loss regimens, as the by-products of weight loss produced by the body may be harmful for the developing baby.

YOUR FREE RESOURCE KIT

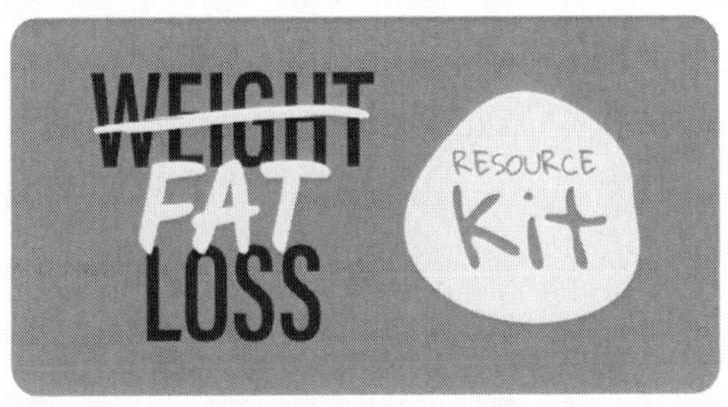

Free Fat Loss Resource Kit

Thank you for the purchase guys! Well, I have a surprise gift here to make the start of this book more exciting and fruitful!

Below this text is a link to the exclusive resource kit which has the recommended products and a progress tracker that will help you track your progress throughout your fat loss journey as you read this book! Isn't that cool! Don't wait and click the link below to claim your free resource material and join my mailing list! Being on the list allows you to be the first to know when I release a new health and fitness book and avail an early bird discount as the book is heavily discounted or available for free for the first 24 hours!

http://leanybean.com/fatlosskit

Happy Reading!

If you find this book useful, please consider leaving a short review on Amazon.

PART ONE
THE HOW

The part where you'll know the shit.

CHAPTER 1
UNDERSTAND HOW WEIGHT LOSS WORKS!

The first thing to understand is that you want to lose that stubborn fat, not just lose any weight! These are two different things. Weight loss can be because of fat loss or muscle mass loss. You want to do the first and avoid the latter.

While our body is completely happy with us getting fat, this sucker is not happy when you are trying to lose it and will give you a hard time doing so. That is because your body is designed for survival mode.

Successful weight loss involves making small changes that you can stick to for a long time. Basically, most of you are not failing at weight loss; you just aren't being able to sustain your diet plan.

CALORIE DEFICIT

Research *consistently* shows calorie intake should be less than the calories burned. It's the single *most important* factor. That's fat loss in a nutshell. It's all about *calorie deficit* really. If someone tells you otherwise, punch them in the face. On top of that, if someone just says do exercise and that's it, break their nose. Those are the people who are responsible for widespread misguidance. Research has supported calorie deficit numerous times! To put it simply...

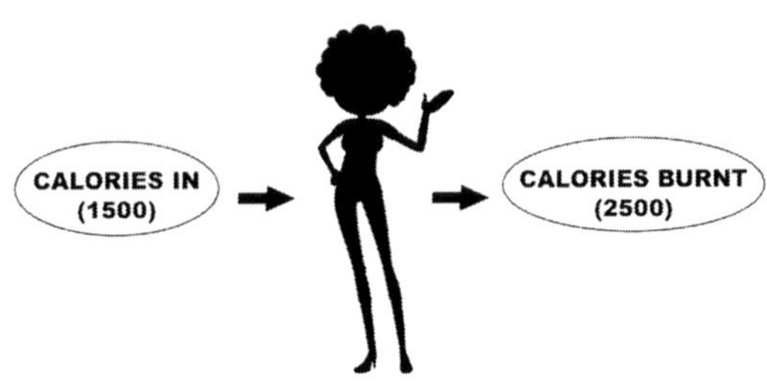

Image 1: Calorie Deficit. *The Golden rule of weight loss*

The Famous Study

Alright, this might seem a little boring, but it is essential to understand and demolish the misguided facts that have been wired into our brains that a certain ratio of macros is what leads to weight loss. Let's discuss this 1964 study[1], which focuses on a group of hundreds of individuals *(precisely 811 participants)* to study the effect of different compositions (ratios) of macronutrients, i.e., carbohydrates, proteins and fats on weight loss. It was done to bust the myths of various macronutrient intake ratios on weight loss; high or low carb or no carb, high or low fat intake and similar protein intake. Individuals were given a fixed number of calories with a fixed *calorie deficit*; the ratios of macronutrients were rotated every few weeks while staying in the same total allowed calories.

They tested it with different compositions such as high carb, low protein, and low fat; high protein, low carb, and low fat; high fat, low protein, and low carb. And other ratios in between while keeping the calorie deficit the *same* across all ratios. What they observed was that all the obese participants lost weight at a *constant rate*. Their study came to the conclusion after tremendous testing that:

> *Reduced-calorie diets result in clinically meaningful weight loss regardless of which macronutrients they emphasize.*

Note: The important thing to consider and take away from this study is, yes, weight was lost but was it purely fat loss? No. There is no doubt that you'll lose pounds on the scale with a caloric deficit of any macronutrient ratio, but the weight you lose on an unbalanced macronutrient ratio is unstable and gained back very fast. Technically you *can* lose weight on a diet of Big Macs, chips, pizza, pasta, etc. if you run on a calorie deficit. However, don't start that because it wouldn't be healthy. To make it sustainable and target fat instead of muscle, we'll be talking about the correct macronutrient ratio in the next coming chapters.

I know it's super tempting to satisfy your palate. You should factor in satisfying foods if you don't want to derail your diet out of dislike for your chosen diet plan.

Making sure your diet is palatable enough to be sustainable is your right. You can make that decision! Hear me out though! This is doable only if you choose healthier options and stay within your calorie limits.

Since the body needs energy to perform its functions and to help you carry out your daily activities, I am by no means asking you to take less calories than the calorie deficit you are already creating. In fact, it is crucial that you consume a sustainable number of calories for weight loss.

When you eat less, your body enters into survival mode as explained earlier, because it starts to believe that it is going through starvation. Therefore, it holds onto your fat stores, which slows your metabolism to balance it with your calorie intake. As a result, you will start to breakdown muscles, which makes you burn fewer calories at rest.

The weight you lose is actually your muscle weight (because you aren't taking enough proteins) and as a result, you lose your body strength and start to fatigue.

CALORIE DENSITY

Let's talk a little about calorie density. You might argue that calories are just calories; well, yes. But we tend to not treat food as calories, which we must. For example, a little bar of chocolate contains way more calories than a large size apple. What we ought to do is eat food with less calories packed in them (in regards to calorie to protein ratio *per* 100 gm of serving). This means more in volume of food while being low in calories.

What's the benefit? These will make you feel full while you're consuming less calories!

A golden tip here would be to avoid unhealthy snacking like chips, chocolates, biscuits, etc. They are not enough to satiate you.

You are going to be a little mad at me when I say that even healthy snacking should be done very, very cautiously. These are the calories that matter most between meals and you must cut down.

To give you a clearer picture, let me show you the real, but absolutely horrid, side of snack time *vs healthy food choice:*

Apple (100 grams): **52 calories**
Peanut Butter M&M's (100 grams): 512 Calories
Hershey's Milk Chocolate (100 grams): 218 Calories
Reese's Peanut Butter Cups (100 grams): 538 Calories
Peanuts (100 grams): 600 Calories
Cashews (100 grams): 553 Calories
Almonds (100 grams): 575 Calories
Walnuts Raw (100 grams): 701 calories
Domino's Hand-tossed Pepperoni Pizza (Medium) 1 Slice: 215 Calories per Slice

Do you see how it blows out of proportion?

This is what happened to a friend of mine who was trying to lose weight for her wedding. She was doing everything right but the numbers on her scale were not budging.

When she discussed this with me as a fellow fitness person, I inquired regarding her diet plan. She would wake up, have her black coffee, have a low calorie breakfast, and then around noon she would have a pack of nuts that she munched on so she could skip lunch and just have dinner.

In her mind, she was skipping a meal! And still not losing. When I sat down and calculated the calories she had during her snack time, it turned out they were even more than a normal lunch meal.

So, she was basically exceeding her daily caloric goal without knowing it and ended up feeling hungrier each day! Because her weight was stuck, the frustration and binges began. Before she knew it, she was off the diet. Blaming her body and metabolism for not being able to help her lose weight.

Next time when you think of having a snack, check its calories first! More on that later.

How much calorie deficit is needed to achieve meaningful weight loss?

This is the first question you will have when you start to think about a diet plan. For most people, setting your daily calorie intake limit to 1,500 calories per day (men) and 1,200 calories per day (women) works completely fine. Another approach is to reduce your calorie intake by 700-1,000 calories per day if you are currently eating over 2,500 calories per day (for both men and women).

This should account for *all the food* you eat between 12 a.m. of the current day and 12 a.m. of the next day. This level of calorie deficit is a good place to start for most individuals.

WHAT WILL HAPPEN WHEN YOU START CUTTING CALORIES

Alright! Let's get down to the nitty gritty now. Our body is designed for survival. Take note! That means when you cut down on calories, your body will start to go into survival mode and slow down your metabolism so that you burn less calories and conserve your stores, and after sometime your body catches up to your deficit (The Halt). What a bummer!

FYI, when you go into that state the first thing that the body breaks down for fuel are your *muscles*. Not fat! Fat comes after that.

This is why it's super important to fulfil your daily protein intake. Our aim is to keep your metabolism active and keep our muscle weight intact! Lean muscles burn more calories at rest due to a higher metabolic rate. Do you get why so many dieticians advocate high protein meals now? Apart from being thermogenic and increasing metabolic rate innately, they will conserve your muscle mass and shift the focus to losing fat instead!

People do not consume adequate proteins by actively supplementing them. As a result, they lose muscle mass, which reflects on the scale as loss of body weight because muscles are made up of proteins. Additionally, they lose energy and start to feel lethargic, which is when your body will go into survival mode.

A big trap that we fall into is just counting calories and not focusing on the macronutrient proportion. This is where you lose! Even if you have cut down your calories and made a successful deficit, it might propel your weight downward but won't sustain it at that number for long. This is because you have to aim for 'fat loss' instead of 'weight loss' for a figure that is more likely to last. For instance, if you have limited your calories but the majority of the calories are coming from fats, then you are surely going to become fat!

Many of you might have already experienced this hard to attain fat loss by now. Trust me, there is a path less traveled that you must take! It is a bit of a hassle and people might call you obsessive, but you have got to really think of what you are putting inside of you instead of just reducing the amount. As I'll be explaining later, there are many variables that factor into fat loss instead of just a caloric deficit, although caloric deficit remains very crucial.

CHAPTER 2
THE UNTOLD FACTS
ABOUT HOW OUR BODY BURNS CALORIES

The secret that I'm about to let you in on proved to be a game changer in my own personal fitness journey. *Understanding how we burn calories!* What actually happens to all the good macros we just talked about taking in? The magic word here is 'METABOLISM'. It is a buzzword too though, I know. You might have seen people who eat up meal after meal and you are so jealous of them not gaining any weight at all. What superpower do they possess? They have a faster working metabolism! You might be asking yourself, "How can I get that too?!" Hold on. Before you get there, let's start with the fundamental knowledge.

Basically, our metabolism consists of four components collectively known as Total Daily Energy Expenditure (TDEE), and these are the buggers that you need to focus on. If you understand this, you have cracked the code to a successful weight loss journey.

Total Daily Energy Expenditure (TDEE), includes BMR, NEAT, EAT and TEF. We'll talk about them in a minute. But first, I want to show you how much each of them contributes to our metabolism.

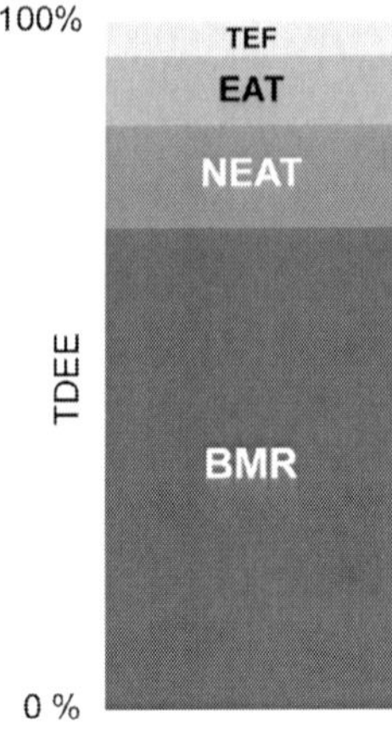

Image 2: Constituents of Metabolism

Brace yourselves for the grand facts:

1. **BMR** ***(Basal Metabolic Rate)*****:** This is the percentage of the calories burned *at rest,* for keeping your system running. Just so that you can *exist!* How lucky! All the reactions going inside of you. The mere pumping of your heart, each breath you take, and many other billions of reactions going on are funded by *60-70% of the calories you eat*. What! 60-70%?! Yes, you heard that right.
2. **NEAT** ***(Non-Exercise Activity Thermogenesis)*****:** It is the activity that we do, other than planned exercise, while we are awake. Everything in

between getting up from bed in the morning and going back to bed at night. For example, walking to your room, eating, doing your day job, walking your dog, doing your chores, etc. It accounts for 20-30% of your calorie expenditure.

3. **EAT *(Exercise Activity Thermogenesis)*:** Now the fun part. This is the *planned* exercise activity that you undertake. Running, jogging, strength training, weightlifting, cardio, yoga, HIIT, etc. You name it. Let me clear your misconceptions regarding exercise. It is widely believed that exercise is vital to weight loss, but how much does it account for the total calorie expenditure? Nobody tells that. It's *only 10-15%*. Let that sink in. All that you have been hearing since the dawn of mankind, do exercise to lose weight. Do cardio or go jogging or run a freaking marathon. Ignoring the simple fact that you have to *control* your *caloric intake*. Kudos to the misplaced priorities, you are still overweight. No wonder. The more you eat, the more you exercise, and it'll still only be 10-15% caloric expenditure of your intake. You cannot out-train your bad diet. Period.
4. **TEF *(Thermic Effect of Food)*:** These are the calories burned while processing and digesting the food you have eaten. It accounts for 5-10%. Proteins have the *highest* thermic effect of food. Meaning, *just* by eating proteins you are burning more calories! Research[1] supports this one also!

This all can be modulated by your diet changes. These facts are the mystery of life unfolded right in front of your eyes. Let me rephrase all the gibberish above:

You're not losing weight because you are eating too much or eating wrong; even when you think you are not!

CHAPTER 3

HOW OUR BODY IS STRUCTURED

Hold your horses as this is going to get even more technical. Let us begin by understanding the first and foremost thing we will be addressing: Our bodies.

To start off, your body is made up of milieu of macronutrients (carbohydrates, fats, proteins), micronutrients (vitamins, minerals), fiber, and water. As their name specifies, they are needed in macro or micro quantities.

As a rule of thumb, a healthy individual who doesn't need to lose weight should be dividing his daily intake as follows:

45–65% of your daily calories from carbs, 10–30% from fats and 20–35% from proteins.

Lets's dive into these components, as their basic understanding is crucial to your weight loss regime.

ROLE OF PROTEINS (MOST IMPORTANT MACRONUTRIENT OF ALL)

First off, protein intake reduces your hunger and promotes satiety! How cool, right? Proteins are proven to lower your hunger. In one study[1] they researched the effects of protein on satiety. Researchers increased protein intake of individuals from 15% to 30% and discovered it increased their satiety level and decreased the caloric intake of the individuals by an average of 441 calories per person because they felt more satiated. *"The satiating effect of proteins."*

This effect of proteins is leveraged in low carb diets as Keto diets because they take less carbs and more proteins. This in turn causes weight loss. However, you go back to square one when you resume your normal carb intake because you didn't account for carbs in your normal day-to-day life.

Carbs are basically the powerhouse of your body, which it cannot live without for long periods. You cannot consume low amounts of carbs for long periods. That's why low carb diets fail to have a long-term effect on fat loss. So, hang in there, buddy! Your body was never designed to go on such diets. It is not you failing at a diet or losing will power, it is just a harmful and impossible way to lose weight for the long-term.

Tidbit: Proteins are made up of amino acids, which are integral to the health of many organs like bones, tissues, skin, hair, and countless enzymes. Basically, they have got their hands in almost all the stuff going on in your body.

Can you eat whey protein?

The short answer would be yes. The long answer is no. Stick with me here. It isn't so black and white. Whey protein is generally safe to take. People take whey protein to fulfil their daily protein goal.

Haven't we all seen those big muscly gym enthusiasts hover over their beloved protein powders as if that was their holy grail. I know the obsession with supplemented protein is sacred!

But as they are taking *only* protein, they tend to develop deficiencies for other nutrients. Compared to the people who take protein from natural sources like meat, yogurt, seafood, etc., they tend to get a ton of other healthy and essential nutrients, which the body needs. Frankly, science has gone only so far with regards to understanding nutrients and our body function.

There are billions of chemical reactions going on in our body every second, all needing different types of nutrients. For this reason, it is way more sensible if you supplement the whey protein intake with multivitamins. The point is that you are missing out on the essential nutrients if you are depending on just the protein powder to do the magic.

Additionally, whey protein might prove to be harmful for those suffering with kidney issues.

Personally, I think choosing organic ways to incorporate protein and nutrients in your diet is the way to go, and I have seen this work wonders on many of my clients and colleagues.

Good Protein Rich Foods to Eat ***(Calories vs Proteins Per 100 gm)***

- Chicken
- BBQ
- Steak
- Meat
- Fish (salmon, tuna or any other)
- Lentils
- Shrimp (Best)
- Prawns
- Greek yogurt
- Cottage cheese
- Eggs (Fried or boiled; fried has fat content because of oil)
- Chickpeas
- Spinach

Note: *Calories vs protein ratio per 100 gm* can vary from one brand or source to another or in one form or another. Always check the ratio for the product you are using.

Also, follow a high protein diet during the duration of your calorie deficit diet till you reach your weight goal. Once you reach your ideal weight, you need to shift your focus on the overall number of calories you are consuming. Keep them in check and there will be no need to go nuts over your protein intake.

CARBOHYDRATES

Understanding that there are *two* types of carbohydrates is important, and both should be incorporated into your weight loss meals.

Just like there are good and bad fats, there are simple and complex carbs.

You might have heard someone say, “use brown sugar instead of white”. Why is that? Simple carbohydrates like white sugar absorb faster, making you feel hungry again faster. Meanwhile, complex carbohydrates are preferred over simple carbohydrates because they are made of longer structures. They tend to take more time to digest, thus providing energy for longer and helping you feel full for longer! This also avoids the sudden sugar rush in blood experienced with simple sugars!

The way your body processes each macronutrient also determines how and which nutrient-dense meals you should be consuming.

When carbs are taken in a correct quantity, and without supplemented sauces and creams, they can’t lead to weight gain. It is better to shift to whole grain diets like brown rice and whole wheat bread to let your body gain enough required fiber!

You do not need to completely cut out carbohydrates from your diet, contrary to popular belief.

Carbs are where most energy of your body is taken from. It's the *powerhouse of the body;* without it you would be dozing off at your workplace and feeling lethargic, which is basically not fun when you are already depriving yourself from all your guilty pleasures. Carbs are full of all good stuff like dietary fiber, which you will need a lot of as we will discuss later.

Carbohydrates Rich Foods

- Whole grains
- Rice
- Sweet potatoes
- Beans
- Legumes
- Quinoa
- Barley
- Starchy vegetables
- Oats (Use raw oats for oatmeal, prepared oatmeal has added sugars)

FATS

Let's take the skeleton out of the closet. Fats are the *energy reserves* of your body. They are not as evil as we have been made to believe. So, are fats good? Let me expand on that. The old maxim of *'excess of everything is bad'* holds true when it comes to fats. Fats are made up of two types of fatty acids. One is essential, which our body doesn't synthesize. The other is non-essential, which can be synthesized by the body. Hence the names. Essential fatty acids need to be taken through diet only, and are extremely important for normal body functions. They cannot be cut out of your diet.

Fats are responsible for providing cushioning to our vital organs like kidneys, liver, heart, and provide insulation to our body. They play a key role in skin and hair health as well. They are responsible for absorption of fat-soluble vitamins. Consider fats as a doorkeeper. If they aren't present, certain vitamins would not be recognized and won't enter the body. Not all fat is bad actually. There are three types of fats that you need to know about:

- Trans fats (bad, should not be consumed)
- Saturated fats (unhealthy, consume with caution)
- Unsaturated fats (healthy, should be consumed)

Trans fats should be removed from your diet or generally be avoided. They are found in margarine, baked goods, fried foods, packaged food, etc. They are added to improve the taste and texture of the food. Even though trans fats have been banned by FDA since 2018, there are still products on the market that might contain trans fats.

Pro Tip: Look for the words *'hydrogenated vegetable oil or fractionated oil'* in the ingredients of the product you are buying. These are basically the fancy terms for *Trans fats*. Even the foods that are marketed as *healthy* might contain some amount of trans fats.

Saturated fats, when taken in excess quantities, increase your cholesterol level. They are found in red meat (pork, lamb, beef) and meat products (sausage, bacon, hamburgers, etc.), chicken skin, butter, ice cream, whole fat dairy products, lard, cheese, pizza, etc.

Unsaturated fats should be encouraged. They are good fats, promote heart health, and lower cholesterol. They are found in fatty fish, nuts, avocados, avocado oil, olives, olive oil, canola oil, spreads labelled as polyunsaturated, soybeans, legumes, grass fed meat, etc. Omega-3 and Omega-6 fatty acids fall under unsaturated fats as well. Sources rich in these fatty acids are an excellent way of getting unsaturated fats.

Approximately 20-35% of calories should come from healthy fat sources for good body function. Unlike other nutrients, where controlling quantities is important, the quality along with quantity control are *equally* important with regards to consuming fats. You should keep track of your fat intake and never set yourself on a goal to completely cut it off otherwise you would be in for a health disaster.

CHAPTER 4
PLANNING YOUR FAT LOSS JOURNEY

Now that we have understood the basic science behind all that happens to the nutrients we take, let's try to apply that knowledge to achieve our goal.

STEP 1
BODY MEASUREMENTS FOR RECORD

You want to know how much of you is fat (and cute).... but wait, how?

These steps are not only going to make you more aware of your body but also be a helpful tool to track your progress over time. There are number of ways to calculate the fat in your body:

1. Body Weight or Body Composition
2. Body Mass Index (BMI)
3. Body Circumference Measurements

1. Body Weight or Body Composition:

The first calculation to note is your current body weight. Simply knowing your weight will serve as a reference point to track your progress. However, if you want to take your fitness game to the next level, having more advanced knowledge and exact know-how of what is going on in your body, then body composition measurement is for you! A normal bathroom scale just tells you your weight. A body composition scale, however, tells you what that total weight is made up of. It will tell you your body fat mass, bone mass, muscle mass, and water percentage individually. It is the best way to know how your fat loss, muscle gain journey is progressing week by week. If you are serious about building and maintaining a fitness lifestyle, I suggest you get yourself a body composition scale! However, a regular bathroom scale would do the basic job as well.

Jot your measurements down and save them in the track sheet provided in the resource kit accompanied by this book. We'll need these figures, bud.

2. BMI:

A commonly used metric in the health industry is BMI; however, it does not differentiate between fat and muscle weight and just tells which weight category you fall in, whether you are *Underweight, Normal, Overweight, or Obese.*

Nonetheless, it's a good idea to know your BMI, because it gives you a base assessment of your body.

So, what is BMI and how do I calculate it?

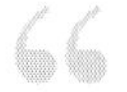

BMI is a measure of body fat based on height and weight that applies to adult men and women.

The resource kit accompanying this book also has built in BMI calculator or you can find BMI calculators through Google. I could write the formula here as well, but it'll cause more work on your part. You can also simply go to a BMI calculator[1] on the Center for Disease Control (CDC) website. I'll share the categories below so that you know what the values are for each category:

BMI Categories:
Underweight = <18.5
Normal weight = 18.5–24.9
Overweight = 25–29.9
Obesity = BMI of 30 or greater

Now you know your BMI category. Kudos to you if you are in the normal *(ideal)* category and want to shed your fat and get lean muscles!

You should know what your ideal weight bracket is. If you stay in it, you are completely fine, no need to go bananas if your weight goes a few pounds up or down while you are already in your ideal weight category! That's why it's important to know your ideal weight category and in which overweight category you fall right now.

3. Body Circumference Measurements:

Next up is Body Circumference Measurements, which records your body size. This method is for your own reference, to track your own progress in terms of size reduction.

Body Circumference Measurement is a basic way to track *fat* by taking girth measurements of different areas of your body, like neck, upper arm, chest, waist, hip, mid-thigh, and calf.

BMI will give you a rough idea and starting point, but if you're daring to dive deeper and want to track your weight loss more efficiently, then this is the way to go as this will give you an idea about your body fat percentage. The testament to this method is that the Body Circumference Measurements method is used by the U.S. Navy.

For men, two measurements are taken: neck and waist. For females, a hip measurement is also taken.

Go ahead and calculate yours. Search for "Body Fat Calculator U.S. Navy" on Google and it'll present you with a list of links to calculators. Fire up a link and calculate your body fat percentage. But again, the values are estimates and not absolute.

I've got my measurements! What now?

Remember the 80/20 principle by Vilfredo Pareto we all hear so often? That's exactly how it is in managing your body outlook as well.

It's **80% Diet** and **20% Workout**.

Yes, you read that right. All backed by science my friend.

Who knew the 80/20 would be so correct when it comes to getting or staying fit?

Are you confused about how diet can be such an integral part for weight loss?

Check out the earlier section where I explained how our metabolism works.

Go read that now you slacker. I know it might be boring, but it is *important*. Think of it as the answer to the mandatory question that your professor loves to put in your exam.

STEP 2
CALCULATE YOUR OWN CALORIE REQUIREMENT

By now you know that it's all a game of calories. Even if you hate math, you'll need to compute these to realize your weight loss dreams! But fear not fellas, I'll be here to guide you step by step through it all. First things first, you need to balance your caloric intake with your calories burned for maintaining your weight and creating a negative calorie-balance or a calorie-deficit for losing fat and weight.

Basal Metabolic Rate (BMR) is the tool used for estimating individual calorie requirements based on the type of physical activities an individual does. Use a BMR calculator[2] or Google *BMR Calculator* and then get the number of calories you need daily. Tada!!

The number you get in BMR (unadjusted for your activity level, actually) is the *minimum caloric intake required* for mere body functioning.

Adjusting the BMR for your activity level

Now that you have calculated the total number of calories needed based on your weight, height, gender, and age, it's time to account for the physical activity you do.

Girl, you can't just laze about and watch Netflix all day while expecting to lose weight magically!

Now, adjust your calories by taking into account your activity level.

<u>Activity Level Explained</u>
Exercise: 15-30 minutes of elevated heart rate activity.
Intense exercise: 45-120 minutes of elevated heart rate activity.
Very intense exercise: 2+ hours of elevated heart rate activity.

To now account for activity, *multiply* the BMR value you got above with the factor mentioned in the following categories that corresponds to your activity level:

Category 1: Little or no exercise (couch potato): **BMR x 1.2** = Total Calorie Need

Category 2: Exercise one to three times per week (somewhat there): **BMR x 1.375** = Total Calorie Need

Category 3: Exercise four to five times per week (you got this!): **BMR x 1.464** = Total Calorie Need

Category 4: Daily exercise or intense exercise three to four times per week (woah! Write me a workout book!): **BMR x 1.55** = Total Calories Need

Category 5: Intense exercise six to seven times per week (you are a pro!): **BMR x 1.725** = Total Calorie Need

Category 6: Very intense exercise daily, or physical job (I don't know why you're reading. Are you testing my knowledge?? *wink*): **BMR x 1.9** = Total Caloric Need

To put that all together. Let's say you are a 30-year-old female with a height of 5 feet 5 inches (165 cm) with a weight of 170 lbs. (77 kg). Based on BMR, your basic required calories (BMR) will be 1,490 calories per day (unadjusted for activity level).

[+ Enter Activity Level]

Let's say you live a sedentary lifestyle, sitting all day in the office with little or no exercise. So, now to account for your physical activity, you fall in the **Category 1** of BMR activity level.

So, multiply 1,490 with 1.2 and this will give you the total required calories needed for each day *adjusted* for your activity level. These are your *maintenance calories*. Which are 1,788 calories per day.

Anything you eat that exceeds those calories based on this activity level, is going to cause you weight gain, and if you eat less calories than those, then it's a deficit, which will help you lose weight. Isn't that simple!

STEP 3
SET YOUR CALORIES AND MACROS GOAL

1. Set Total Calorie Intake

Your goal for meaningful fat loss should be an intake of 1,500 calories per day for men and 1,200 per day for women (if your *maintenance calories* are at or under 2,500 calories per day).

If your maintenance calories are more than 2,500 calories, say 2,600 calories, then create a deficit of 700 to 1,000 calories. In this case, you should be eating between 1,600-1,900 calories per day for both men and women. But always keep a fixed calorie deficit throughout your diet. Say if you want to create a deficit of 1,000 calories, then stick to it throughout your diet journey. The higher the deficit, the higher the rate of fat loss. But the deficit should not be more than 1,000 calories per day.

2. Set Macros Ratio

What should be the ratio of macronutrients per your daily calorie intake?

Ideally it should be
40:30:30
Carbs : Fats : Proteins

You should aim to have 40% of your calories come from carbohydrates, 30% from fats and 30% from proteins of your total calories.

This is the *ideal* ratio for diet as explained earlier as well.

But realistically an average person who doesn't want to go nuts over their weight loss should be able to maintain *at least*:

50:30:20
Carbs : Fats : Proteins

At least 50% of your calories should come from carbohydrates, 30% from fats and 20% from proteins of your total calories.

3. Convert Ratios into Grams

For a 1,500 calories per day diet with a ratio of 40:30:30, the following grams of macros are needed:

Carbohydrates: 150 grams
Fats: 50 grams
Proteins: 112.5 grams

But, how to convert ratios into grams?

First you need to calculate *calories* from each macro ratio. Say, we want to consume 1,500 calories per day with a 40:30:30 ratio of macros. For this diet, macros should have the following calories:

Carbs 40%: 600 calories
Fats 30%: 450 calories
Proteins 30%: 450 calories

Now convert these calories of each macros into grams:

Carbs 40%: 600 calories/4 = 150 grams
Fats 30%: 450 calories/9 = 50 grams
Proteins 30%: 450 calories/4 = 112.5 grams

Conversion Note:
Carbohydrates= 4 calories per gram
Fats= 9 calories per gram
Proteins= 4 calories per gram

What Is The Amount of Protein You Need to Take?

There are two methods to calculate your protein needed:

1. By body weight: Protein intake should be between 0.7-1 grams of proteins per pound of body weight. It should be no less than 0.7 grams per pound of body weight. You can go up to 1.5 grams if you add intense exercise in your daily routine.

2. By diet ratio: Say you need to consume 1,500 calories per day in 40:30:30 ratio: 30% of 1,500 is 450 Calories.

The 450 Calories should come from the proteins as per diet ratio. Generally, 1 gram of protein has four calories in it. So, 450/4 gives you 112.5 grams of protein which you need to eat daily.

I would suggest you follow the second method, by diet ratio, for your required protein.

STEP 4
FOOD PLANNING

Let's discuss the most common questions regarding food planning first. I get asked questions on the topics I mention in this step most commonly and it makes sense to address them here.

Type of Meals

Carbs or no carbs? No need to cut carbs off the list. Just focus on overall calorie and macronutrients targets for each day.

Selection of Food

While selecting your meals, you need to qualify the food based on only two factors. If it passes. Go for it! Otherwise steer clear.

The first factor is knowing the calories vs proteins in your meal. Basically, what you need to look for is calorie to protein ratio *per* 100 grams of what you are eating. You want to go for the food that gives you more proteins in *less* calories *per 100 grams*. This will allow you to achieve your daily protein goal while consuming less calories. The following example will clarify this first factor:

- Shrimp: 99 calories for 24g proteins (per 100 grams per serving)
- Meat: 143 calories for 26g of proteins (per 100 grams per serving)

- Chicken: 239 calories for 27g proteins (per 100 grams per serving)

If you have a choice of these three meals and you want to have more proteins but less calories, then shrimp is the way to go.

Tip: Divide proteins in grams by number of calories. You'll get the percentage of protein content for given calories. Continuing with the above example:

- Shrimp: 24/99= 24% Protein
- Meat: 26/143= 18% Protein
- Chicken: 27/239=11% Protein

That's how you verify the proper selection of your food! Choose the one with minimum calories but highest protein content in it.

The second factor, the likeability of the meal. Above all else, you should enjoy yourself through your weight loss regimen, otherwise you won't be able to stick to it and it will fail like everyone else's.

Numbers of Meals

One of the most common questions I receive is about how many meals to eat each day. It doesn't matter how many meals you have or when you eat, whether you take three large meals or six small meals in a day. Have the number of meals you are comfortable with. However, if you divide your allowed calories among small meals and spread them out throughout the day, like six meals a day, you'll feel less hungry.

If you have a large appetite, then go for three to four big meals per day. That way you'll have a large quantity to eat in every meal and will satiate your hunger more. Divide total calories allowed among the number of meals you want to have.

Timing of Meals

Timing is only important if you have workouts to incorporate. You should eat 30-45 minutes before or after the workout if you haven't eaten in hours. That's it. Make your life simple!

Next thing you might be thinking is when you should eat your protein when you are working out? The answer is you don't need to go nuts over taking proteins within 30 or 40 minutes post workout. This time window is referred to as the *anabolic window*. Research has shown that the anabolic window lasts for 24 hours. If you can take protein within 30-40 minutes post workout, then do. If you can't, no worries.

Meal Planning

Planning is the keyword here. For example:

- Plan 'go-to' meals. They will be your life savers when you don't have time or cannot go into unchartered waters.
- Plan your 'all day meals', what you'll be having and at what time of the day while considering your allowed calorie limit.
- Choose foods that are less calorie dense. All natural or unprocessed foods are less calorie

dense and are more filling. Fast foods and snacks pack very high calories and are not filling, which makes you tend to eat more, exceeding your allowed calorie limit.
- Keep in mind what you like and dislike. Plan your meals around them to achieve a long-term and sustainable adherence to the diet.

STEP 5
HOW TO KNOW THAT CALORIES OF WHAT YOU EAT

The single most important factor, which is going to be the most vital to your weight loss journey, is measuring the calories of what you eat.

Weigh what you eat! If you plan to do only one thing in your life regarding fitness, this should be it!

Buy a kitchen scale, whichever kind fits your budget. You don't need to go over the top. Buy one that is readable and is able to hold the cups, bowls, plates that you want to measure in and has a flat weighing surface.

The testimony to the benefit of this method are the results produced that I have personally witnessed for other people and myself.

When I first started to measure my food on a weighing scale and log it into a food tracking app (more about that in the next section), I admit it was cumbersome. But I had completely stopped eating the food supplied at the hospital cafe and instead started packing my own weighed and calculated lunches and dinners if I had a long shift. People around me would call me anal and restrictive, they resented me for not indulging in the midnight cookie after a hard day at work. After all, it is just a cookie to reward yourself. But trust me, being in tune with what I put inside me and doing the cumbersome task of math was a gateway to understanding how inaccurate I was on the calories I was consuming in my previous yo-yo diets.

Many have made weighing food part of their eating lifestyle now. It is only a task initially, but after doing this for a few weeks, you tend to know the calories of the food you eat regularly and are just in tune with the kind of calories you are consuming.

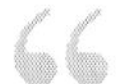

> *The magic tool – a food scale.*

The key idea to take away from all this is that you can eat everything (healthy), just in the right macro ratio and calorie portions.

Remember our aim is to feel full throughout the day while staying in your new calorie window.

Knowing how many calories you consume is the cornerstone of your fat loss plan. The main cause of us getting fat or not shedding fat is underestimating or misreporting our calorie intake as it has been mentioned earlier in the book while discussing snack calories.

In fact, one study[3] looked into this and found out that even dieticians tend to misreport their food intake by an average of 223 calories, with some underestimating their calorie intake as high as 800 calories, and others as low as 300 calories. And the case for the general public is much worse.

- A Big Mac has a whopping 550 calories. You wouldn't even feel that you have eaten that many calories and if it's a Big Mac meal that's 1,100 calories. *Ouch*!
- A slice of regular sized pizza has somewhere 200-300 calories.
- A biscuit has 25 calories. Eating four biscuits costs you 100 calories.
- A date has 75 calories. Yes, that small tiny date!
- The nuts you have on your table, 100 grams of those guys throughout the day will cost you 660 calories. But who considers it eating?

When we are munching here and there mindlessly on these supposedly tiny guys without knowing how many calories you eat in addition to your breakfast, lunch, and dinner, and it's not even a proper meal. That's where all of us lose.

Normal meals are less calorie dense and are more filling, which keeps you satiated with less calories while delivering all the healthy and essential nutrients.

STEP 6
HOW TO KEEP TRACK OF YOUR PROGRESS

Now that we have all that out of the way, you may be asking how do you keep your protein and calories in check?

Well, it's pretty simple but people might see you as a crazy scientist when you do it. You'll have to just deal with it because that's the most crucial element. Without it, you cannot keep your protein and calories in check.

This simple yet crucial element is checking for calories and protein for every food you eat. Log your food in a food tracking app on your smartphone by searching the name of the food or by scanning the barcode. You must do this every time you eat something. Every F****** time. *Literally.* Whether it is a full meal or just one biscuit. Just log it in. LOG. IT. IN.

For packaged food, scan the barcode to log ingredients, proteins, and calories. You can also manually enter the ingredients of the meal and it will give you the total calories of that meal. Essentially a meal's calorie value is the sum of all its individual ingredients' calories. Water contains no calories, FYI. Drink plenty of water; it will keep you satiated as well. Take note of that! Keep track of your daily water intake as well.

How to Track Your Calories and Intake

I have used a number of smartphone applications for this purpose. Every app is lacking in some aspect. By far the app that has given me exceptional value and covered all my needs is MyFitnessPal by Under Armour. This has become the go-to app for the cult trainers and professionals. An app is the pivot point of this diet plan.

Setup your calories and macro ratio in your app that we discussed earlier.

What is MyFitnessPal:

- USDA-verified nutritional stats of thousands of foods.
- Enter the ingredients individually for a meal in the app to see a cumulative sum of its calories if you don't find its name.
- It also suggests recipes on what you can make or eat with their exact nutritional values. This helps you know what you are eating and where you stand at your daily goal! You can plan your whole week ahead.
- Log what you have eaten into the app (name of the food) and the quantity (grams). Indicate which meal it is: breakfast, lunch, dinner, etc. to keep track.
- The app will tell you how many carbohydrates, proteins, and fats you have consumed (paid feature). In the free version it will only tell you about the number of calories you have taken. To have full control and information on your diet, the paid version is necessary.
- You can make your own custom recipe, which are meals you make yourself. You just need to put in the ingredients per 100 gram serving and save it if you make it frequently so that it is easier to enter next time. For example, you make your own recipe of scrambled eggs, which varies due to ingredients like number of eggs, butter or amount of oil used. Make your own recipe and save it once and for all! Next

time just pull up the saved recipe if you have eaten it!

- Check the calories of foods and snacks by scanning them in app to track calorie intake.
- Since understanding the app is not the aim of this book, I suggest you watch a tutorial on how to use MyFitnessPal app or any other app that does the same functions so that you can understand and use the app efficiently.

Track Your Calories:

Log in your current day's calories till 12 a.m. midnight. After that, the next day starts. Follow this strictly. No carry over calorie-deficit to the next day.

Track Your Weight:

You should be well aware of how your weight is performing. Tracking your weight is one of the important measures of progress.

How to weigh?

Weigh yourself on a digital scale in the same place daily, naked after using the washroom, and before breakfast.

Now, you might be wondering, how many pounds should you be losing per week?

Losing two pounds per week is easily achievable and recommended. Over the course of the week, adjust your calorie deficit in a way that you lose two pounds per week. Losing more than that might affect your energy levels. A person weighing 250 lbs., for instance, will lose more pounds per week than a 165 lb. person, which is totally normal. A heavier man could probably lose up to 3.5 lbs. while a less heavy man will lose two lbs. per week. The more fat you have the faster it starts to shed! It is a normal thing under the same calorie deficit. You get the idea.

Weekly average

Take weekly averages instead of relying on daily weight numbers. This is more accurate because your weight fluctuates on a daily basis. To get the weekly average, divide the sum of seven days' worth of your daily weight by seven. You should always look at the *weekly average* to see your progress because daily weights fluctuate and can be misleading and discouraging! For women, menstruation causes high fluctuation in weight. For the days during menstruation, continue to track weekly and *compare monthly*. Use the progress tracker given with this book to keep record and track your weight throughout your journey.

Weekly Progress Pictures:

Find a spot that has good light where you can take pictures every week. Make sure that the environment and lighting of that area is consistent across all your photos, which will help you notice the changes in your body. Keep your body relaxed and always take photos in the same relaxed posture for the best comparison. Take front and sideways pictures, and if possible, then back also. Take and log in the progress picture in the app with date and weight. Don't forget to wear your undergarments for this one. After all, it's going on the cloud buddy! Save them securely on the phone, just in case.

The First Seven Days

For the first week eat your normal diet that you already do. Monitor and observe your *current* calorie intake for a week by weighing your food and logging the calories of the quantity you eat in the app. Weigh and log everything you eat. I mean everything, literally. Even the single nut you have eaten. Just note and observe. I challenge you to do it for one week. It will give you insight into how many calories you are consuming daily. Compare that to your calorie requirement (discussed previously) and see how far off you are. After a week, see your current calorie intake that you are taking, create a calorie deficit of about 1,000 or cap your maximum calories to 1,500 or 1,200 per day for men and women respectively.

Pro-Tip: If you decide to go to a restaurant, plan ahead. Decide what you'll have and calculate the calories if the menu doesn't state them or ask the chef about the ingredients and their quantity so that you can enter them in your app.

CHAPTER 5
HOW TO EAT THE RIGHT QUANTITY

Portion Size vs. Serving Size

Many people confuse portion size with serving size.When you turn over a packaged product, there is some information regarding the *serving size*. The serving size is a set standard. For example, a cup of instant noodles contains one serving, which contains 240 calories. But what if you were to take less than one cup. How would you count the calories then?

And what's portion size? Well this one is under your control, it is a choice you make for example if let's say Mr. X decides to eat more veggies in a day on routine, he is increasing his portion size for veggies. There is no estimate of calories provided in this way.

Instead a more accurate way is to weigh your food and put it in a plate. Now that is your chosen portion size you can count your calories for.

For example, you put a bowl of oatmeal on the weighing scale and it indicates 45 grams. Now check online for the number of calories in 45 grams of oatmeal. Log this in your diary and you are done.

When you keep doing this as part of your routine, you are likely to learn by experience the serving size and associated calories.

Pro Tip: Opt for a sugar free or low calorie or fat free version of the same thing when available. This will greatly allow you to enjoy that food while saving on calories also!

Kickstart Your Day!

Below are some examples that you can add into your breakfast diet routine. These are quick and easy ones that can help you plan your meals by having a quick short and sweet list:

- Eggs (in any form)
- Steak
- Sandwiches: Mustard sauce, patty, salad of your liking, egg boiled, tomatoes, capsicum, onion, whole wheat bread. Whole wheat bread has more protein content than brown or bran bread and it is organic with no artificial sugars. Just make your own flavor and stay away from mayonnaise, ranch, thousand islands, spreads, etc. You can use *mustard sauce* because it doesn't contain any calories. Other spreads and sauces are packed with ginormous calories. Keep track of the calories, using the app, for the individual

ingredients based on the quantity used in your recipe. It'll give you the total calories of your sandwich. You can save it as your *custom recipe* with all the nutritional details in the app for future use as well.

Pro-Tip: Bake your sandwich! Preheat the oven to 160° C. Bake it in the oven for eight to nine minutes. It'll get roasted, making your sandwich crispy and tastier. It was my go-to breakfast meal!

- Greek Yogurt: It has particularly high protein content! Add fresh fruits like strawberries, etc. Watch out for strawberry *sorbet*! It has A LOT of sugar, which is bad! Try adding brown sugar, raisins, almonds, crushed peanuts, Use 10 grams daily. Mainly vitamin C and calcium should be looked out for. Almonds fulfil your Recommended Daily Allowance (RDA) of vitamin C. Greek yogurt and eggs are excellent sources of calcium.
- Grilled Fish (or however you like to make fish. Grilled fish just tastes better)

Good Example Add-Ons for Your Recipes:

- mustard sauce for flavoring your sandwiches, burgers, or steaks
- cucumber
- tomatoes
- broccoli
- cauliflower

- cabbage
- capsicum/bell pepper

Avoid add-ons that contain lots of sugar.

You get the idea. Plan your breakfast; this list will give you an idea what kind of breakfast you should go for. There is no hard and fast rule. Test what suits your routine and palate and keep your main two goals for the day in-check:

1. allowed daily calorie intake

2. required daily protein

That's it!

CHAPTER 6

HOW TO TAME YOUR HUNGER

AND FEEL FULL LONGER

Drink one cup of coffee (240 ml) two to three hours after breakfast or after any of your meals. Not before. Otherwise it messes up the absorption of iron and other minerals like iron, calcium, magnesium and vitamin D from your gut.

You can drink another cup at lunch or dinner time; or after them, whichever you prefer while staying in your allowed calorie window.

You can drink a maximum of two cups of coffee in a day, no more than that. Better to stay at two cups though. One cup of coffee will provide around 200 calories but depends on your personal choice of coffee. So do not exceed two cups so that you can have enough calories left to cover your proteins.

Frequency of meals doesn't matter. Do what suits you. If five or six small meals suit you, go for it. If three large meals is how you want it, do it. Just stay within your allowed calorie limit. Be sure to at least eat three meals.

Fad Diets!

Now that we have all that discussed, let's talk about why you must take the high road and choose a sustainable diet rather than the quick solution!

We have all heard the words "fad diets" thrown around in health podcasts or nutrition articles, but what exactly does a fad diet mean? It essentially is cutting down on one or more food groups, mostly carbs or fat, completely from the diet. These diets will tell you that you will lose weight faster but will come with a strict set of life bending rules that will leave you tired and frustrated at best.

I know! It's tempting when the weight loss is promised to be this fast, but we all know that if it was supposed to be working these many wonders, each one of us would be fit and having our dream beach bodies sunbathing on an island right now.

Apart from them having higher chances to fail due to non-compliance, fad diets also make you gain weight back faster and more than you ever had initially. Not to mention the health catastrophes like hair loss, skin sagging, and so much more that follow. You don't need to cut any food group for fat loss! You can eat what you like while staying in the criteria we set.

Most fad diets will have you starving, which will result in an intake of less protein. When your body faces a deficit of the protein and amino acids that it needs, it will turn towards itself and start breaking your muscle down. There you go! Instead of losing fat, now you are losing proteins!

Fad diets are basically like painting over a dented car, instead of going to the source and repairing the dent. It will only be a quick fix that will put you into a perpetual diet state. Whenever you leave that diet you will be gaining those pounds or possibly more back. The goal is to devise a healthy meal habit that puts you in a calorie deficit even after having completed your daily nutritional requirement.

Carbohydrates are the main source of energy for the body! You cannot stop eating this group. If you do so, whenever you eat them again, you'll gain weight as fast as you lost. Fad diets cause deleterious effects on health and lead to greater weight gain in the long-term.

Crash diets! Oh my! Where do I start?! For starters, they are not even effective because if you are taking in more fat content and not taking required proteins, the body starts to store fat. Weight will be lost but it will be muscle weight that is shed and you'll start to feel less energetic. Whenever you resume to normal eating, you'll get fat again.

Keto diet is a waste. Studies[1] have shown numerous times that it helps you lose weight initially, but it's not long-term. Research[2] has shown it is not sustainable and is not a lifestyle solution. Studies have found that no significant weight loss occurs in the long-term. While marketing and numerous books on this regime are spreading like a pandemic, the truth is, people need to steer clear of them if they want a long-term, sustained weight loss solution.

I eat salad; don't tell me it's not safe either!

Well, salad is safe, but its toppings, not so much. Watch out for the toppings! Mayonnaise, cheese, etc. Try to eat salad alone and avoid these add-ons! Caesar salad has 250-400 calories! Watch out, mate. Trust me you can do much, much better by using those calories correctly. One tablespoon of mayonnaise has *94 calories*! Imagine pouring two tablespoons of mayonnaise in your daily diet. That's almost 200 calories out of the window!

PART TWO
THE HELP

Weightlifting? Cardio? Swimming? Yoga? What the hell!

CHAPTER 7
MYTH BUSTING

There's a lot of misconception around exercise and weight loss. Although planned exercise along with a calorie deficit does increase fat loss, but it doesn't happen with just any exercise like many presume. In fact, I see people doing the wrong exercise all the time and then they wonder why they aren't shedding any weight. Many of the people that have come to me seeking diet advice even consider standing for a long time a huge caloric burning activity. They then complain, saying, "All my work is standing and I still do not lose weight." Why is that you may ask? Let's clear all these misconceptions so that we can differentiate myth from the truth when it comes to exercise and fat loss.

Dilemma One: To Exercise or Not to Exercise?

Research[1] has proven that the most effective way to lose fat with a calorie deficit diet is to opt for *strength/resistance training* and NOT cardio. Why is that? Well, the answer would be ‘muscle mass’. Resistance training, along with good protein intake, will *build* your muscles. While cardio will surely help to lose weight, but at the expense of losing your muscles.

The magic recipe here is *lean muscle mass*.

If you are on a calorie deficit without any protein supplementation, you are going to lose muscle mass along with the fat. But isn’t losing fat the whole deal? Well yeah it is, but it isn’t so fun when your fat loss journey begins and halts soon just because you have lost all your essential BMR!

On the contrary, increasing lean muscle mass will increase your basal (resting) metabolic rate *(BMR)* and you’ll burn more calories for just doing nothing (because muscles burn more calories at rest, remember).

If protein supplementation is good for your BMR, imagine what amazing benefits an exercise that's proven to increase muscle mass could do! Resistance training will do just that!

To explain this in a more science backed way, a study[2] was conducted looking specifically at this and it came to the conclusion that when you lose fat purely driven only by calorie deficit, your body’s muscle building rate drops 27%, while if you add *resistance exercise* along with a calorie deficit, your muscle building rate returns to normal.

Interestingly, if you supplement your calorie deficit with *proteins* along with *resistance exercise,* muscle building *increases 34% above normal levels!* This is responsible for gaining lean muscles and preservation of muscle mass and resultantly increases BMR as already explained above.

You see, protein intake plays the most vital role in helping you lose weight out of all other macros.

According to another study conducted in 2012 on obesity, they found that over the span of a year, the people who were on diet-only interventions lost 8.5% of their weight, while only 2.4% was lost by the exercise-only participants.

But the group which combined both diet and exercise lost the most, that is *10.2%* of body weight.

CHAPTER 8

DO LIGHT ACTIVITY – BUT WHICH?

CARDIO? STRENGTH TRAINING? HIIT?

The addition of exercise points toward the fact that you should be focusing at least twenty minutes of your day on resistance exercise.

TRX is a particularly good to be done at home. Why? Well because it is easy, convenient and the results it delivers makes it my personal favorite! It is suspension training. How it works is that it acts on deep and core muscles to increase body strength and builds up those muscles while simultaneously correcting body posture! Killing two birds with a stone!

TRX doesn't only help build core body strength, but also gives shape to the body very efficiently which we all desire. I remember when I first started doing TRX at the gym, I basically could only continue it for three months due to my hectic hospital schedules, and yet its effect lasted a long time even after I left it. It didn't just maintain my body posture and the core muscle strength, but also my body shape all along. While the effects of doing weightlifting goes away way sooner, like in months once you stop lifting weights. Strength training that involves your whole limb or core muscles is the way to go!

To get more optimized results, try using a workout app that assists you in targeting specific body areas, like upper limb, lower limb, etc. It'll help you target areas by selecting the region you want to focus on and plans and guide your workout by compiling a group of exercises needed to achieve that goal along with the time and repetitions needed. It shows you the right way of doing the specific exercise with sample video clips, which helps to attain the correct posture during the exercise to engage the muscles and avoid problems associated with wrong posture. I have personally used the Fitify app for this and it serves the purpose really. You could give that a try or find an app that suits you!

Also install a full-length mirror in your work out space, it doesn't just help you take amazing gram-worthy gym selfies, but also allows you to self-correct your posture while you're working out.

So, is cardio any good?

First, let's look at what cardio is.

Cardio is also known as aerobic exercise because it utilizes your body's oxygen and elevates your heart rate. It is considered an athletic exercise, which is designed to increase body activity, health of heart, and induce an overall positive effect on the mental and physical state of your body. But they are *not* the right exercise for fat loss because their main focus is mobility and activity.

Stop cardio! Yes, you read that right. The first exercise that might come to your mind to aid your fat loss journey will be cardio. But that is not the case in reality. Cardio sends the body into a catabolic state and it breaks down muscle along with fat, the former of which you want to conserve in the first place! Conversely, resistance and strength training conserves and builds lean muscles. More muscles = more BMR, meaning when you have more muscle mass, you start to burn more calories while you rest.

To put things in perspective, American Council on Exercise states that a 120 lb. person will burn 11.4 calories per minute by running (cardio), which means for a 10-minute run, that person will *only* burn 114 calories. That means cardio is more time and energy consuming compared to resistance training. This is because cardio focuses on deriving energy from glycogen stores in muscles. It has an overall negative impact on lean muscle mass let alone build muscles!

But it doesn't mean you must steer clear of cardio at all times. In fact you can go for cardio to maintain weight after you have achieved your desired weight and have returned to your normal caloric consumption. More about how to do that at the end.

Does standing for hours count as exercise?

I hear people say this all the time! That they stand a lot due to their nature of work, so they don't need any more exercise.

Truth is there is just a *marginal* difference between the calories burned while standing as compared to sitting. Standing not only makes you tired but isn't burning as many calories as you imagine.

On top of that, standing isn't even contributing to any muscle building. You have to opt for *planned exercise* instead of just depending on a menial number of calories that you burn standing.

As discussed earlier, adding at least a 20-minute resistance training session to your daily routine will do wonders to your muscle building and caloric expenditure.

If you are a more active person and prefer cardio as exercise, then you should go for High Intensity Interval Training, HIIT. A good example of that is a sprint. This is where you do a 30 second burst of a run with all your energy or till you burn out, then take a break for a minute or so (recovery period), and start your sprint again. This is a kind of interval training that focuses on short bursts of high energy followed by a recovery phase. It will make your body derive its energy expenditure from *fat stores* which makes it a good form of cardio for fat loss.

PART THREE
THE HALT

The shit that scares you.

CHAPTER 9
WHY IT HAPPENS AND HOW TO BREAK IT

Expect the halt, it is bound to happen on your journey to fitness. But do not be discouraged. Consider it a speed bump instead of a road block!

Basically, the halt is a plateau that occurs because there's no more *calorie deficit*. You have already lost body weight, which has decreased your BMR (slower metabolism) because a smaller body burns *fewer* calories. For this reason exactly it is important to supplement your body with proteins because it builds muscles and increases lean body mass, which in turn increases your BMR, and voila! Now you will burn more calories even with a smaller body! Also, *when* the halt happens may vary depending on your initial macronutrient proportions. For example, Sam has 20% body fat while Leah has 10% before they start their deficit diet. Leah is more likely to reach a plateau sooner than Sam.

When you are on a caloric deficit diet, your body catches up and adjusts to the number of calories you are taking so that you don't lose any more fat. To overturn and rotate that homeostat of your body, you must add protein and increase your calorie deficit further by decreasing the number of calories you consume or increasing the exercise activity.

This phase shouldn't bother you until six to eight weeks after you have been into your fat loss journey. If you have reached that phase, pay careful attention to the following factors because most of the time, they are the biggest culprits.

1. Salt!

Let's talk about why the sudden jump on the weighing scale happens. A major reason for this is the common household item we all deem very innocent. The sodium in the salt retains water in your body that can show up on the scale as weight gain, when in fact it is just water weight and not fat gain. To avoid this inconvenience, try steering clear of food items that are loaded with salt. Check to see if you have been taking more salt lately. Make sure you are comparing weekly averages of your weight and comparing weekly photos of your progress.

Recent researches have also shown that salt can *increase* hunger by creating resistance to a hormone called leptin, which is responsible for making us feel full.

2. Sugar!

As mentioned earlier, white poison, oh, I mean sugar is a very fast burning carbohydrate. Even if all other factors are kept ideal and sugar intake is not controlled, this can lead to weight gain! Notice if you have lately started taking more sugars in any form. Whether it is in your drinks or in the form of desserts. Sugar slows down weight loss momentum. If you need to have sugar in your coffee or tea, switch to brown sugar. It is a healthier and a far better option than white sugar.

3. Caloric burn

When in halt, try to get out of it by either further reducing your calories by 5-10%. Or you could amp up on the exercise and burn more calories to give your metabolism a push out of the halt. Just because your weight isn't moving doesn't mean you are not losing fat. You might also not be losing weight if you are new to weight training, because in the start you build muscle and lose fat at the same time, which looks like you are at a plateau. Results will become apparent in three to six weeks because there comes a time when your body can't build muscle as fast as the weight loss. That's when you start to see your weight go down on the scale.

4. Period (for females)

During your period, your appetite changes, making you crave sugary and high calorie foods, which may affect your calorie deficit. On the other hand, even if you maintained a 1,000-calorie deficit during this time, hormonal changes could cause water retention. If you weigh yourself during this time, chances are that you will start thinking that your diet is not working. For this reason, you should track your weight weekly but compare your progress *monthly*. You should measure your weight on the last day of your menstrual flow every month for comparison.

5. Stress

Take a chill pill! If you are under stress, your body produces cortisol, which is a stress hormone that may convert your food into fat instead of energy, cause water retention, or signals the body to hold onto fat. Try something that can help you relieve that stress. I would personally write a journal, paint, or simply just go out for a walk/run, or have a cup of coffee (black of course) by myself. Find your own little stress buster!

6- Alcohol

Basically, consumption of alcohol will slow down all other digestion processes that help so many micronutrients get absorbed. It will alter your digestion such that your body will prioritize flushing out 'harmful by-products' of alcohol instead of targeting and breaking down your fat stores, even if you are in caloric deficit while you are consuming alcohol.

6. Health Issues

Sometimes you are trying your best and you are still unable to lose weight. You are leaving no stone unturned, but the scale is refusing to budge?

If you're doing everything that has already been said in this book but are still failing, it's time that you take a deeper look into your health. There are many health conditions that affect body metabolism in a negative way, of which include diseases like hypothyroidism, polycystic ovarian disease commonly known as PCOS, and also menopause in women.

7. Maintenance Phase

Well, if you have tried everything that has been mentioned so far but that stubborn weight is still not coming off, it is highly likely that you have now come to a state where your body has caught up and isn't letting you lose more fat because it sees it as an attack on the survival instinct on the body.

Now it's time where you must stop the caloric deficit and instead calculate your maintenance calories and shift to them for about *two weeks*. This signals to your body that you are out of the survival mode and basically it should shut off its ninja-style protection against weight loss. Your body eases hormones and the body system returns to normal during this period. After two weeks start again with your diet plan. This will reset your system and give you the same weight loss momentum that you initially had when you first started on this diet. Don't freak out yet! You won't gain back the weight you lost. You will just be aiming to maintain it. It's basically a system reset.

After you have successfully tricked your body for two weeks into a normal body calorie intake, now you may start creating the deficit you were in again! It may seem funny but it really is like a restart and restores your body to default settings to make your machinery work at its best again!

Also, isn't it a well-deserved and fun break, aka mini vacay from the pursuit of weight loss, while your body prepares to get itself on track to achieve new goals!

CHAPTER 10
BREAKING BAD HABITS

Don't fall trap to the following bad habits as they are subtle and not really noticed if you aren't critically analyzing your diet plan. Break these bad habits to be more efficient in your diet management journey!

- Advice: Do not drink your calories. Try sticking to water. If you do have a drink with calories, you must restrict it to under 120 calories.
- Do not eat while watching the news, a TV series, or movies. When watching something, people tend to forget the portion they need to eat and binge more often when engaged.
- Be mindful of what you are eating when you sit with your plate of food. Give it the attention you would to your spouse really! This trick makes you feel fuller and appreciate what you are having.

- Do not go on binges when in the car. Make it a rule to not eat in the car. Tell yourself that you will have whatever fits your daily diet when you are out of the car seat.
- Surround yourself with people who have similar fitness and health goals. It makes you feel like you're a part of a good thing, keeps you motivated, and causes less distractions from your diet plan.
- Keep healthy snack options in your favorite snack places.

CHAPTER 11
FOODS TO WATCH OUT FOR

Watch out for the before dinner snacks as you get home!

While you might enjoy the little munching of these snacks while the dinner is being readied, you'll be surprised (shocked actually) how many calories they include. Just log them in and your eyes might pop out. Somctimes it is equivalent to a *full blown meal.*

Some foods weigh less but have gigantic numbers of calories. For example:

- refined foods, which are packed with high calories and very low satiety index
- mayonnaise
- dates
- chips

- nuts
- peanut butter
- fast food. You can have fast food, but it eats away your allowed calorie limit. For example, a McDonald's burger will cost you somewhere around 700 calories. This doesn't even cover your protein needs and you are almost halfway through your calorie window. You can stay alive on Big Macs if you stay within your calorie window, but it won't be healthy, and you'll start losing your body energy because you'll be shedding your muscles.
- junk food
- snacks (snacks and Netflix gotta stop!)
- white sugar! White sugar is a very fast-burning carbohydrate, meaning it absorbs fast in the body. It makes you feel hungry faster. Instead of using white sugar, switch to brown sugar, which absorbs slowly because it's organic. White sugar makes the blood glucose level rise very quickly. On top of that, if you eat desserts or sweet dishes after your meal, it overloads your body with sugar and sends it into a sugar shock. Excess glucose, which is not required by the body, starts to store in the body as *fat*. Also, more sugar intake will make your weight halt or plateau and your scale won't budge. Sugar interferes with the protein you consume as well, making you burn less calories than what you should! Help yourself and switch to brown sugar!

All in all, it's all about managing your allowed calorie limit and always, always fulfilling your protein intake. You can taste stuff and eat a bit, but not to an extent where it is affecting your macros, caloric, and protein intake.

CHAPTER 12
TWO ABSOLUTE RULES TO ABIDE BY

If you only follow two things from this book, they would be the ones mentioned below. All of the people who I have helped achieve their weight loss goals always abide by these two rules! Consider breaking them as the eighth cardinal sin. That's how crucial it is for your weight loss plan.

1. Complete your daily protein intake goal. No matter what. Plan your meals and eat those foods that help you to achieve this goal.
2. Consume the allowed daily calories within 12 a.m. of the current day and 12 a.m. of the next day. No carrying over of calories to the next day. No living on more calorie-deficit than required. Period.

Eat meals that contain everything, but your main focus will be these two guys, proteins and calories.

But wait, what about the leftover calories from the current or previous day?

Never transfer your leftover calories to the next day; 12 a.m. is the time when your day starts or ends. If you have leftover calories from the day, consume them before 12 a.m. Enjoy them with anything you like while staying in your calorie window! But never transfer them into the next day. Strictly. STRICTLY. And never go on to the next day with more calorie deficit than is required.

THE DIET AFTER DIET

HOW TO GET BACK TO YOUR NORMAL CALORIE INTAKE

Now that you have reached your goal weight, the next thing to focus on is how do you get back to normal calorie intake? Do you have to stay in this caloric deficit forever to maintain our body? The good news is *no*.

You can bump up to your maintenance calories over the span of a few weeks. But a sudden increase will lead to weight gain. You must let your body adjust to the increase in calories or your body will consider it a 'surplus' and store it as fat!

You need to increase 100 calories per week till you reach your recommended required calories for the weight you wish to maintain. In this way, you will be eliminating the calorie deficit and entering maintenance calorie phase.

In case you want to be on the safer side, increase your calorie intake by 50 calories per week. Gradually increasing your calories allows your body and hormones to absorb the increased energy and utilize it for the body instead of considering it as an extra and storing it as fat. During the fat loss period, your body has been reset to lower calorie intake. Any sudden increase in calorie will be seen as an excess than what is needed by the body. So, you have to transition your body into the maintenance calories slowly to make it beneficial! Once you get to the maintenance calories, you'll stay in the achieved weight till the time you start to consume more calories than needed by the body.

CONCLUSION

The aim of this book is to help you achieve weight loss by targeting *fat* instead of other important components of your body; to let you break the mentality of "I CAN'T" and reach "I WILL".

When you put this book down, you should be able to look at food as energy and nutrition that is required to run your body. Food that is palatable and pleasurable is a plus of course. The point of this book is not to demonize food, it is to know when and what to eat. It is an important decision, just like other important decisions we make in our life. Isn't what you're putting inside of your body just as important and should not be taken so nonchalantly? For now, try analyzing where you are in your journey to fitness and carry on with the advice and guidelines that were provided in this book.

ONE LAST THING...

Every year people around the world make many resolutions and lists to achieve, and it wouldn't be false if we were to say that the most ardently made resolution is to stay fit, lose weight and improve health. This book was written with just that in mind, to help you achieve and actualize those goals and promises that you made to yourself.

If you enjoyed this book and you think people can benefit from it please share it with others and leave a review so that the reader community is confident in picking the right book to kickstart their fitness journey.

In leaving a review, you help the community take a step towards their goals and our shared experience can perpetuate into becoming a mass fitness and health boost. Also, when you share with people something of value, people associate that value with you. As it is the book that helps them but just because you shared the book, people will associate that value and that feeling of gratitude with you. It is an easy and authentic way to build your personality profile while you end up helping others along the way.

- Dr. Maria H.

Leave a Review

PAIR THIS BOOK WITH THE JOURNAL!

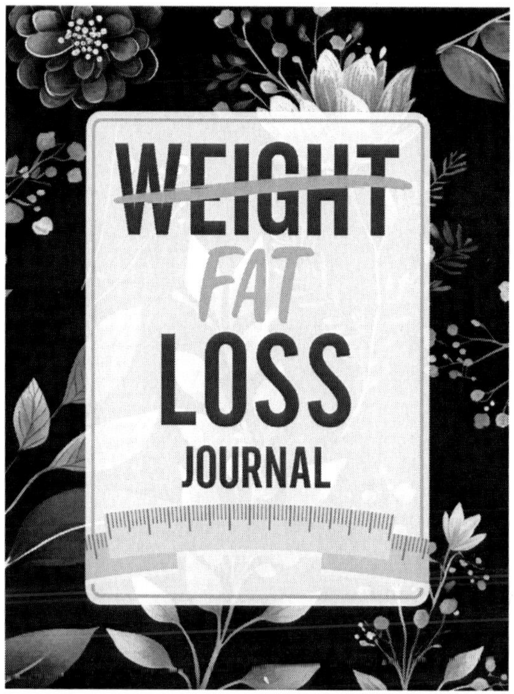

Get on Amazon!

Our beautifully illustrated Food & Fitness Journal is designed to help you track what you eat, prepare diet plans, monitor your fasting, develop healthy habits, and reach your fitness goals.

It Includes:

- Daily food log

- Daily fitness log
- Daily calorie tracker
- Daily feelings and emotions tracker
- Complete weight tracker
- Complete measurement tracker
- Water intake tracker
- Steps log
- Sleep log
- Caffeine log
- Weekly and daily goal setting, and plenty of space for notes

Our hope is that this journal will inspire you to adopt a lasting lifestyle of healthy eating and regular exercise. We welcome any feedback you may have and look forward to hearing from you.

Share your progress with me!

fatloss@leanybean.com

Got any questions? Fire me an email!

dr.maria@leanybean.com

ENDNOTES

1. UNDERSTAND HOW WEIGHT LOSS WORKS!

1. https://pubmed.ncbi.nlm.nih.gov/19246357/

2. THE UNTOLD FACTS

1. https://www.ncbi.nlm.nih.gov/pmc/articles/PMC4258944/

3. HOW OUR BODY IS STRUCTURED

1. https://pubmed.ncbi.nlm.nih.gov/16002798/

4. PLANNING YOUR FAT LOSS JOURNEY

1. https://www.cdc.gov/healthyweight/assessing/bmi/adult_bmi/english_bmi_calculator/bmi_calculator.html
2. https://www.calculator.net/bmr-calculator.html
3. https://weightology.net/do-dietitians-accurately-report-their-food-intake/

6. HOW TO TAME YOUR HUNGER

1. https://pubmed.ncbi.nlm.nih.gov/16476868/
2. https://www.ncbi.nlm.nih.gov/pmc/articles/PMC4990387/

7. MYTH BUSTING

1. https://pubmed.ncbi.nlm.nih.gov/9280173/
2. https://journals.physiology.org/doi/full/10.1152/ajpendo.00590.2013

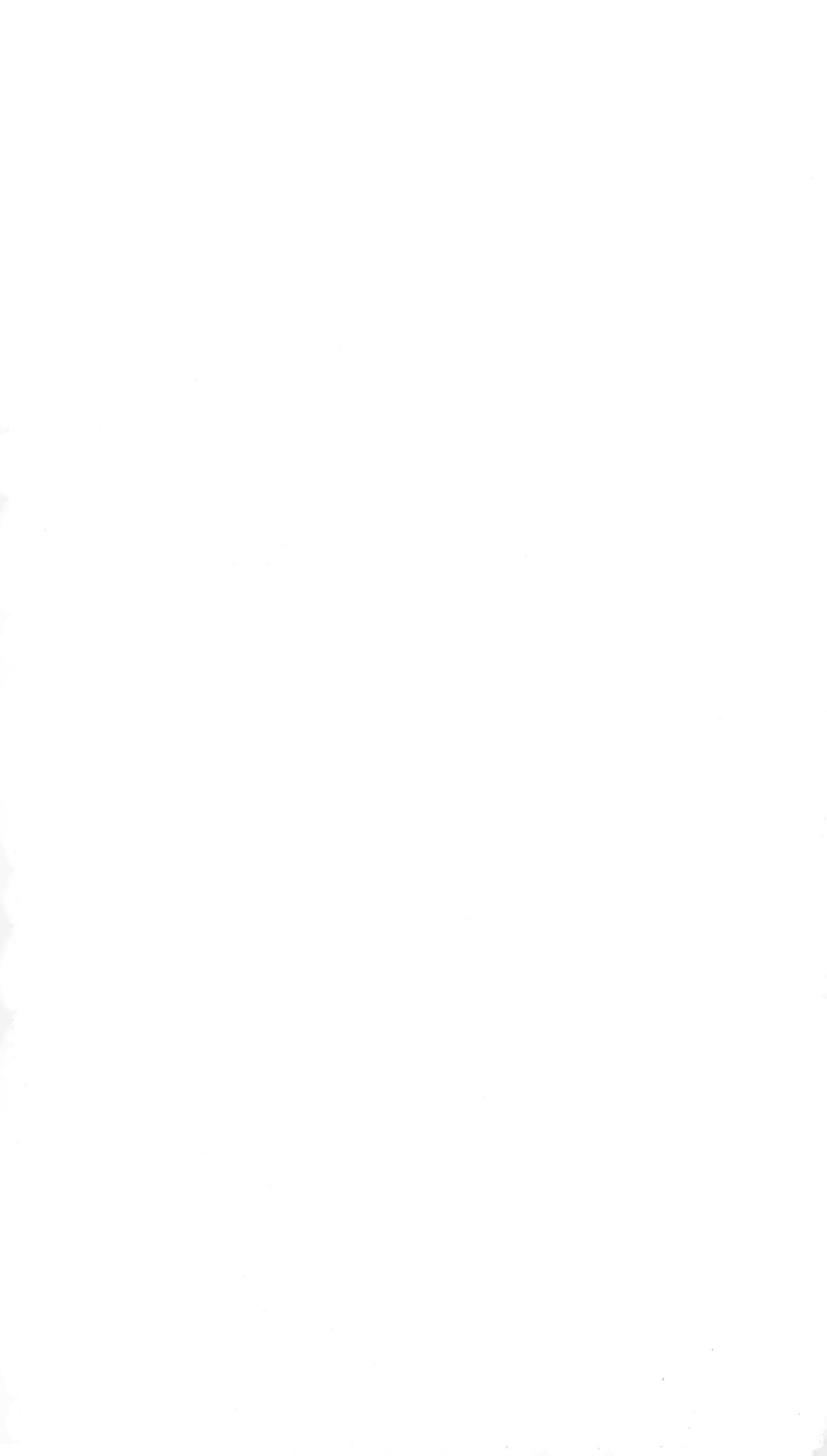

Made in United States
North Haven, CT
29 April 2023

36020492R00069